COMM

Transform Your Body and Your Life With the Power

of Yes

By Paul S. Boynton

Except when an individual's complete name is used, people mentioned in this book are fictitious composite characters intended to illustrate specific issues and situations.

Publisher

Toby Dog Media

http://tobydogmedia.com

Cover Design

Paul Brand

Manuscript Design

Craig A. Hart

http://www.craigahart.com

This book is dedicated to the "Begin with Yes" Facebook family. You inspire me every day as you commit to live meaningful, joyful, love-filled lives. I am touched by your willingness to support and encourage each other. I am amazed at the challenges you have faced, the dreams you are making come true, and your tenacity and willingness to step up and step out—to keep moving even when you're discouraged, afraid and weary. You are my heroes and this book is for you!

Acknowledgments

This book would not have come into being had it not been for my dear friends, the co-founders of the GENAVIX Network, Mike and Tricia Benton. After years of stress and work, I found myself needing to make major changes to improve my health. Mike and Tricia invited me to experience their *90-Day Commit To Get Fit* program. I agreed and was amazed by the positive progress I made in such a short time. During the process, they asked me to write a book for fitness that would incorporate the style and principles from my first book, *Begin With Yes*. Since I felt such a deep connection with their gentle, one-step-at-a-time program, I agreed to do it someday. They persisted in asking me about this book when I would see them in the gym. I am glad they did because that someday is now. I have no doubt that this book will find its way into the hands of many people who need to believe that they can feel good again, and I'm grateful to Mike and Tricia for the part they played in making it a reality.

My dear friend, confidant and fellow author Jacob Nordby served as the structural development editor for this book. He helped me pull the whole thing together and organize my thoughts from start to finish. Jacob has his own great tale of physical transformation, which is why I knew that he would bring a deeper level of understanding to this project. Jacob is living proof that the principles of *Begin With Yes* and this book are true. I'm grateful that he pulled the yoke along with me until this book was finished all the way to the end.

Artist and writer Barb Black lent her superior skills as grammarian and proofing editor to this project.

Craig Hart, author of *Becoming Moon* and other books, handled the manuscript design and ebook conversion.

I want to thank my children, including their spouses and my grandchildren—who love me despite my imperfections and continue to laugh at my jokes, allowing me to think I'm funnier than I really am. I bet I love you more than even I know and certainly much more than you can imagine.

And finally, thanks to Michael who knows I march to a drum that even I can't always hear. He and Toby keep me grounded and smiling and always happy to head home at the end of the day!

Foreword

We all desire to pay better attention to our health, yet we seem to take care of everyone and everything else before we take care of ourselves. We wish to change but often lack a clear vision of how to get started. In the past, managing our health by reclaiming the power of personal choice was never a topic for public discussion. This is still true, but an unhealthy lifestyle catches up to us in many ways. Our ability to enjoy life because we are physically and mentally healthy is not the only thing at risk. We now need to understand that our financial wellbeing is deeply affected by whether or not we are healthy. Since we are all required to carry insurance now, the only way to reduce our personal healthcare cost is to stay healthy or participate in our plan's prevention program or corporate wellness programs.

The Affordable Care Act of 2010 allows companies to incentivize employees and their families to improve health risk factors through proper nutrition, exercise, stress management and lifestyle change. For the first time in our country, we can reduce healthcare costs by submitting our health risk factors. These discounts can be as much as 30% for those employers who choose to offer such incentives. But as we all know, making the commitment and staying the course is not always easy.

We live in a world where mass media is used to promote health and wellbeing, yet tempts the consumer with highly processed, refined, genetically modified, unhealthy foods. The fitness industry chains and home fitness equipment providers prey on our desires to be more active through discounts and low cost memberships with the promises of support and results. In reality, this model is based on the hopes that you never show up but that you also never cancel. Once the home purchase is made, the provider is simply a marketing company that no longer cares about the proper use or value of its product to the consumer. Giant food companies, fitness chains and home fitness providers employ the mass media to confuse the consumer with far-fetched health and activity promises to push sales. As a result, we are faced with a growing national obesity problem, despite extensive scientific research that exercise and proper nutrition are good medicine.

It can be overwhelming to think about how the deck is stacked against us, but we have not crossed a point of no return. The good news is that your health and wellbeing are in your control. No matter how bad you feel you can change! Understanding where and how to find the right support within the community and alongside your friends and family are key elements for success. The first step in solving a problem is in the acknowledging that you have one. Change in our country occurs faster and more pervasively when we are impacted financially. Yes, we all vote with our wallets. This is also true when it comes to healthy choices and a more pervasive selection of food and services. With education and personal commitment to change, we can achieve optimal health and well being by effecting change where we live, work and play. The growth of Whole Foods, Trader Joe's and Organic farming are examples of national movements, but don't discount your local grocers, full service health club, and local restaurants. They too will offer healthier and less expensive choices if the demand is created and value is received. We all have a part but it all starts with education prior to making our purchases. Proper nutrition and an active life style neutralizes stress. Gaining the knowledge of what is and is not a proper diet, combined with finding the foods you like to eat and exercise you like to do significantly increases your likelihood for success. The fitness industry is much broader than the franchise chains and the home market providers. There are many community-based providers that are individually owned and have a large stake within the communities they serve.

Our foundation and experience is within this part of the fitness industry; we realized many years ago that our industry only addressed one of the four pillars necessary for obtaining optimal health—exercise. Nutrition, stress management and ultimately behavior modification are just as important, but were non-existent disciplines within our industry. Exercise is very important but education, individual nutrition and life style customization are equally required for optimal health.

With knowledge comes power and this is also true when one commits to achieving and sustaining good health and well-being. The proper attitude, knowledge and action—in that order—are truly all that is needed for success. You would never step on the field to play football with a baseball glove. You position yourself to win by first understanding the game you're in and coming equipped to play! Deciding to live a healthier lifestyle is no different. We must understand the rules, come equipped, learn the fundamentals…and of course practice!

It was for this reason we created the GENAVIX Wellness Network™. Under a common brand, the Network consists of independently owned, full service health club facilities that offer preventative care and wellness services in support of improving our population health in the communities we serve.

Each owner collaborates and pledges to provide the same pervasive Wellness assessments, programs and services, known as Healthy*CARE*™. These programs and services are community-based and are delivered by certified Wellness Coaches, Registered Dieticians and other trained professionals. For the first time within our industry our Network offers outcome-based services and programs that do not require the purchase or commitment of a monthly membership. All of our programs and service focus on initial outcome then sustained outcomes through assessments and individual wellness plans that are customized for the individual based on achievable goals. We discovered over the past five years, the key elements for success are in little rather than big steps to achieve behavior change.

As a network it is our mission to *"To provide wellness solutions that result in lifelong health and personal transformation."* We want everyone to understand that they have not passed the point of no return and that it is not too late to experience amazing health, and in the process save money and enjoy life more abundantly. This book embodies our voice as a network to provide the education, motivation and support to everyone willing to take the first step on their journey. It is our deepest hope as a Network that we can impact our own industry and partner with healthcare, and insurance industries.

Paul Boynton became our client a few years ago. Shortly after meeting Paul, we read his first book, *Begin With Yes*. We immediately knew that he held a big missing piece of the puzzle for people who want to make real changes. There is something about the way he leads people through a gentle process of conversation to uncover their real dreams and hidden fears—it is simple but powerful. He does not dump a lot of platitudes on his readers or expect them to believe his ideas. Instead, he gets right into the heart of the issues that have been holding people back. Then he offers practical guidance for how to address them one step at a time. Over and over again, Paul says, *"Don't believe me. Put these ideas to the test. They work every time they are used."* When we read his words, we knew that we needed Paul to write a book specifically about health and wellness and how one can take the first step towards transformation no matter your age, size, gender or race.

Like those of us in the GENAVIX Wellness Network, Paul has a deep belief and passion to help people who have given up the hope of feeling healthy or good about themselves. We hold that hope for them until they are ready to hold it for themselves again. The way we do this is by providing the guidance and coaching to take their first step. We also know that wellness is about community—surrounding ourselves with likeminded people who are on a similar journey. Paul addresses these things in this book in ways that are easy to understand and implement.

The book you are holding in your hands provides the first steps into living a life of better health. We are proud to have seen the need for Paul's newest book and are honored to have been part of his own journey to health and well-being. We urge you to read this book and give Paul the opportunity to show you how to begin your journey of great health. Let's start today!

Mike & Tricia Benton
Co-Founders, GENAVIX Wellness Network™

Introduction

Fitness. It's a powerful word and used to market everything from cars and sporty clothes, to pills and protein powders—and more. But isn't it funny that, when it comes to fitness, many of us don't feel at all powerful?

Many people feel discouraged and perhaps even ashamed of their bodies as they are bombarded with constant images of beautifully muscled people with tanned skin and big, white smiles. They feel like these must be the lucky few with the right genes or born under the right stars, but that they themselves must struggle along never feeling great about themselves. They assume that to get physically healthy and feel vibrant would be a hero's journey, and, to be quite honest about it, they aren't sure they have the necessary energy to get the job done.

I want to offer this gentle conversation as a way to change this perception, and I invite you to join me as we can unpack the beliefs and fears that have blocked so many of us in the past, and the begin moving toward the dream we have for our health and our bodies.

I believe that all major change begins in the mind. Whether we want to build a skyscraper, take on a whole new career, or move to a new part of the country, nothing happens until we begin to imagine what we want.

The problem with "major change" however, is that...it's major. For example, if you have a lot of weight to lose, or it has been years since you touched your toes, you may feel that it's more of a challenge than you're up to.

This book is different because, although I want to help you imagine the best body and health you could desire, what's most important to me is that we begin from where you are standing (or sitting) right now.

I want to have this virtual conversation with you and acknowledge your skepticism and your fears, along with your hopes, and your needs.

After you read this book, my desire is that you will see your own body with greater love and appreciation. I want you to be drawn forward into what you want most in a way that inspires you with possibility rather than shame or competition.

And I want this to be a journey that will last the rest of your life and be filled with joy and wonderful experiences—not just be a short, obsessive sprint that leaves you disappointed and exhausted.

If that sounds good, are you ready to begin?

Lao Tzu, a Chinese mystic and philosopher from ancient times whose Tao Te Ching was written about 2,700 years ago and has deeply affected the world since, is credited with the famous saying

"A journey of a thousand miles begins with a single step."

For many of us, the idea of getting our bodies healthy and fit may seem like that kind of journey. This little book is designed to help you begin where all journeys must—with the first step.

Let's Begin

People sure are worried about their health these days. We have skyrocketing healthcare costs, obesity rates that are higher than ever in history, and many degenerative diseases that are tied directly to a lack of fitness. Compound that with an absolute avalanche of advertising and messages from the media about how we should be a different size and shape— and lifestyles that are busier and more stressful than ever.

It's a funny thing, this modern world of ours. We humans have worked so hard for many, many centuries to create a civilization with plenty of food, good roads, safe drinking water, and lots of machines to do our heavy lifting, but somehow that hasn't translated to healthy, vibrant bodies for many of us. What should be a natural, well-balanced life because of our systems and computers and machines has actually become more stressful.

Researchers have found that stress is a major contributing

factor that plays into many of the illnesses we so dread, like cancer and heart disease. You would think that with all of the conveniences we have built to reduce wear and tear on our bodies, we would be living with low stress. That's simply not the case. In fact, people living in first world countries are shown to experience the highest stress levels of all.

We lead busy lives that make it easier to eat fast food, work long hours in a sitting position, after which we race home to fall on the couch for a few hours before going to bed, only to start all over the next day. By the time the weekend comes, most of us are so weary that the idea of going outside or to the gym for healthy exercise seems like just too much.

Now comes the mental and emotional part: not only do we have a hard time fitting everything in and taking good care of ourselves, there's a constant drumbeat from the media about how much better we should be doing—which adds to our guilt and stress. Our bodies feel sick and heavy, and we feel badly that we are not doing enough about it.

This is specifically what I want to address.

Our bodies are meant to last for a lifetime and feel good. Doesn't that have a nice ring to it? I want this book to pop a big stress bubble for all of us and get us moving in ways that help us return to our natural state of health and joy.

Almost no one lives in the same house all of their lives, but all of us live in just this one body. Like a home that you would clean and repair and furnish with beautiful things, we want to revive our sense of how to really treasure our own bodies. Deepak Chopra wrote, *"If we are creating ourselves all the time, then it is never too late to begin creating the bodies we want instead of the ones we mistakenly assume we are stuck with."* And that would be a good mantra as we begin to make positive changes in how we feel and look.

Now, this book is meant to be simple and was written to support or complement one of the many fitness plans already available to you. I chose a program called "Commit To Get Fit", which was offered by my local gym. It was a great program for me because it required me to stretch, but is also grounded in reality. It included a huge educational component, acknowledging the realities of my busy life, and included an emphasis on healthy eating along with a healthy exercise program. I hope you have already chosen a plan that you can follow as you get ready to commit to making positive changes in your life. Having worked with people for so long, I have learned that the biggest barrier we have to achieving what we really want is lodged in our minds.

As I did in the mechanics of *Begin With Yes*, I frame this book as a conversation so that together we can acknowledge and gently remove those obstacles, allowing us to move forward with confidence. I'm not going to beat you over the head with more of the same information you already have on your bookshelf. But believe with all your heart that this conversation will get you through the sometimes excruciating first steps of commitment, and keep you moving forward until your goals have been achieved.

This book won't have recipes or specific exercise regimens.

We will do some exercises, though. I want to help you get in touch with your natural desire for a body filled with good energy, good feelings, and good health that you will want to go all the way through with whatever program you choose as a structure for your fitness plan. We are going to have a chat about who you are, what you want, and how to connect with that in ways that get you moving for good.

I'm ready to get started, but I have to be honest. I have tried a lot of times. Even though I lost weight and felt better for awhile, I always ended up back here. Why is this time going to be different? I want to do this, but I'm not sure I can handle another failure.

I'm so glad you were able to say that. We need to have a sort of contract at this point to be completely honest with each other. You started off exactly right with this question. Thank you.

In return, I'll be honest with you. I can't force you to change, but can promise that this time will be different if we get to your real desires and the root causes of why your previous efforts haven't stuck long term.

I don't want you to get started on yet another journey that you just can't finish. Instead I want to help you to go into the unconscious side of this question and find some of those invisible reasons why your past commitments have wavered, and why things haven't worked before.

Commit! is about drawing a new line in the sand and stepping over it into the journey. But wait, before we make any commitments or step anywhere, let's pause, shall we? I don't want you to make any decisions or take any actions before you are ready.

Maybe you know someone who has gone shopping for a big ticket item. If they met the wrong salesperson who didn't take time to learn their needs, but relied on charisma and high pressure to make a deal, they probably got home later and contracted a bad case of buyer's remorse. If they couldn't return the item or get out of the deal, perhaps they found themselves stuck with a car, or furniture, or some other expensive reminder of a hasty decision. I don't want you to be motivated by my reasons, the media's reasons, or by society's, either.

The only way this will be a sustainable journey of transformation is if you take the time to know yourself and your true desires—your very own reasons why.

As we continue this conversation, I intend to ask you more questions that will not only help you unearth the reasons you really want this change, but also discover the reasons it hasn't worked before. The good news is, you can do something about those things, and when you do, it will make the rest of your adventure feel a lot lighter. Who wants a long, rugged trek for the rest of their lives? Not me, and I suspect not you, either.

One other thing I want to share with you is a phrase they use in Alcoholics Anonymous and many other recovery groups and self-help groups: "Progress, not perfection".

In other words, we want to set you up for success, not another disappointment. Part of that will need to include falling in love with the process of change. We are constantly sold on end results but never on the journey to get there—especially if that is a long one and requires the best of us to get there. As a result, when we don't drop three pant sizes or develop lean, muscular abs in time for our beach vacation, it's easy to get discouraged and jump back into our old ways of eating and non-exercise.

For that reason, I want you to fall in love with your own progress. I want you to fall in love with the body you're living in right now, and then keep loving it as it changes according to what you wish to see. After you have achieved an impressive transformation, I want you to feel tremendously comfortable in that new skin.

One of my friends was a personal trainer. He coached clients through exactly this process over and over again. He once told me that some of his students went all the way. They lost a lot of weight and built up their muscles until they could easily qualify to appear in fitness magazine photos. I asked him what happened after that.

He said, "You know, many of them made permanent changes and went on to enjoy their new fit, active lifestyles; however, not just a few didn't know where to go after they climbed that mountain. In the absence of a big goal, they slipped back into their old ways and a year or two later, I'd see them at the store and they would avoid me because they had gained back the weight."

So, as we continue this conversation, I want to help you establish the reasons that will help you get all the way through the process and then have sustainable reasons to permanently keep the routines and supportive nutritional habits in your life.

Good news! You don't have to be a strong-willed person or already have a disciplined mind to get started. This process will work no matter where you are right now.

So, you're saying that even if I have tried and failed, or don't have a lot of confidence in my own strength to follow through, this could still work? Sounds too good to be true.

That's right. Now, I promised to be honest with you, so here goes. Jillian Michaels, one of the star trainers on the *Biggest Loser* TV show said, "Will is a skill." I won't pretend that you don't need willpower or focus or determination to make this change. You do.

Will is a lot like your muscles. It can be developed and strengthened. You don't have to start out with bulging will-muscles. When you make the real choice to commit, you are already exercising your will. The more you make choices toward what you want, the stronger and clearer your will becomes. For example, in surprisingly short time, you'll be able to attend a party where they are serving all sorts of food that would once have been your Achilles Heel and you will know exactly how to handle the situation. In fact, it will become more and more like a game.

Remember Bill Murray in the movie *What About Bob?* It involved a successful psychotherapist who almost loses his mind after Bob, one of his most dependent patients, a manipulative, obsessively compulsive narcissist, tracks him down during his family vacation in hopes of finding relief. His exasperated therapist had to help him learn to take ridiculously small actions that would help him be able to have a more normal life.

One of the memorable scenes in the movie is when the Bob is stuck in the lobby and can't move in any direction. Dr. Leo Marvin finally comes up with a phrase that acts as Bob's key—"baby steps".

Bob begins repeating his mantra over and over again as he inches forward into motion, "...baby step onto the elevator... baby step into the elevator... I'm *in* the elevator. Ahhhh!"

That may make you chuckle if you remember the movie, but it's what I'm suggesting here. When you start to break down the whole process into its individual steps, the choices don't seem so daunting, and you don't need much willpower to accomplish them.

Here's a question to ponder.

"What are three examples in my life of how I naturally use my will power?"

I encourage you to sit down for five minutes and write these down, then think about them.

In my coaching work I often find that people who are feeling stuck tend to globalize their frustrations. In other words, they take the experience they are having in one area and paint the whole sky of their life with that brush. When we take the time to untangle the threads a bit, the truth comes out that they aren't incompetent, depressed, or failing in every single aspect. In fact, they usually get excited to discover how many ways they are performing at above average levels.

This is about getting clear, accessing our personal power, and taking inspired action. We usually get that formula backwards, though. We see someone else accomplishing great things and try to duplicate their action. Because we haven't laid the other critical foundation stones, of course we don't see their results—ignoring the work, effort and time that led to their success. Then we unfavorably compare ourselves to them and assume that we just aren't "one of the lucky ones".

As we continue together, I will invite you to slow down and gently lay those foundation stones that will support you for the rest of your life.

Now that you say it that way, I can see how often I have tried something before but haven't been clear about what I really want. Instead I just use other people's goals or successes as my road map. That hasn't been working, but I am not sure how to find those hidden obstacles and strengths that are relevant to me. How should I begin to do that?

That's a great question. Let's dig in here, shall we? I'm going to ask you to go get a notebook and pen for this part. Don't worry if you aren't great at writing. This isn't for anyone else to read and most of what you'll need to write will be short. The reason it is important to write these down is because the act of putting it on paper gets it all outside your head so you can see them. These "hidden obstacles and strengths" have been living in your head for a long time and it is nearly impossible to focus on them. They are hiding in plain sight, too. You will be surprised by how obvious some of them seem, but isn't that the way big stuff reveals itself?

Okay, I'm going to stretch and breathe for a minute while you find that notebook.

Have it now?

Great.

Start at the top of the page and write these words: *My Body Is…*

Underneath that, write the first things that come to mind. Don't worry about saying something right or phrasing it positively. Just write the things you might never say out loud but hear inside your head. Remember, this isn't a test—it's a mirror. We just want to see what is really there.

How did that go?

Now read those words out loud beginning each sentence with "My body is…".

How do you feel about what you just said?

If someone else walked up to you on the street and said them to you, how would you feel?

Are they honest?
Are they harsh?
Are they set-in-stone truth?
Did you use sugar coating?

See, when you make a statement like "I am ____" or "you are ____" or "my body is ____", your subconscious mind accepts it as fact. There's little wiggle room. Your subconscious mind observes and records your feelings and words like a court reporter. Your conscious, thinking mind is another story, though.

If you have been reading some of the inspiring positive books out there, you may have learned to use affirmations to reprogram your subconscious mind. I love affirmations, but I also want to help you line up your actions and results with your highest truth.

Even though our subconscious mind's job is to record and translate our thoughts and feelings into reality, most people don't realize that if they are constantly saying things that aren't true, they set up a situation that psychologists call "cognitive dissonance". Your conscious, thinking mind spots the lie and says, *"Hey! Wait a minute. That's not true."* Then it gets into a wrestling match with the subconscious. We want our conscious mind and subconscious to work together—not fight each other. Because if the conscious and subconscious are at war, we will have a much harder time getting what we want. So, we want to consistently use powerful, honest communication with ourselves which will integrate what our rational mind can believe and our subconscious mind will put to work behind the scenes to help us achieve those dreams.

We will get into how to use what is called **powerful self talk** later. Getting this right will make you feel like you have learned real magic. Teaching your conscious and subconscious to speak the same truth about who you are, what you want, and what you are doing about it makes the whole process an exciting dance.

This is making a lot of sense, but I know there's more to the story with me. It can't all be subconscious mind stuff and self talk, can it?

You're right. That's just one piece of the puzzle. I started there because it is the biggest, most important part. There's more to that one and I'll give you some more work to do in that area as we go.

Let's talk about beliefs—those things we accept as true about ourselves and about life in general.

It's such a huge topic that sometimes it's easier to start with some simple lists. These will help give you clarity on your core beliefs.

Still have that notebook handy?

Start a new page and write this:

My Top Five Physical Accomplishments So Far

Underneath that, write anything that comes to mind that falls under the category of physical achievement. That can include anything from "ran a marathon fifteen years ago" to "beat cancer last year" to "lost ten pounds before Christmas", or anything else. Nothing is too large or small here.

Please be sure that you don't add a "but" after the accomplishment, though. What I mean by this is that most people diminish or disregard their accomplishments by saying, "but I took six hours to run the marathon" or "but I gained back fifteen pounds".

Don't worry, we'll give you room to be honest about your disappointments soon. For now write at least five things that represent an accomplishment—even if some of them don't seem too impressive. If you have more than five that show up immediately, write them all down. Some people find that they have a long list of achievements they haven't paid much attention to, so this is time to get them down on paper.

After you have written them down, please read them out loud to yourself. Do you know what we're doing with this? It's called anchoring. When you write it down and read it out loud, you are beginning to anchor something in your mind and body.

Next, write a new heading:

My Five Biggest Physical Disappointments So Far

Some of these might be obvious, such as, "gained sixty pounds during pregnancy and haven't lost the weight yet" or "hurt my back at work and can't run or lift weights like I used to".

You might be surprised to notice something really old like losing a race at school or being called fat by someone who mattered to you. These things carry a lot of energy and, if we don't let them come up, they can act as perennial saboteurs in our psyche—always weighing us down on invisible levels when we set out to change our lives.

I encourage you to allow just a little time for this part. Especially let yourself feel what you're feeling with these things. We won't linger here too long, but it's so important to unburden yourself from these hidden weights.

I asked you to write down disappointments in the Physical category, but if something shows up as a big sore spot in another area, please write it down. I have seen many people change their lives very quickly after they acknowledge a major pain or wound that seems unrelated to the particular goal they are working on at the moment.

My dear friend Jacob packed on over seventy pounds that he struggled with for over fifteen years. He tried all the fad diets, did extreme exercise in spurts, and even ordered weight loss pills. He yo-yoed up and down, sometimes losing thirty or forty pounds, but always gaining back the weight. He was discouraged and was fairly sure that he would never get back to his ideal weight. The day came when he was able to find and acknowledge some deep old disappointments that seemed to have nothing to do with physical weight. Shortly after this, he made a big commitment to his health, lost all the weight within a year and now wears the same pant size he wore in high school. He told me that the journey was not only worth it, but also couldn't have happened if he hadn't looked at the other issues in his life.

This section isn't meant to replace therapy. If you discover issues that are a lot bigger than writing a few lines in your notebook, I encourage you to find a professional who can help you deal with them. The time you spend here can be priceless to your long-term success and happiness.

For now, after you have written at least five things in your notebook, please review them. Feel what comes up as you do this. Afterward, please say "thank you" to yourself out loud. This is important work you're doing. Many people aren't courageous enough to do it, but you are. Because that's true, I want to thank you, too.

By the way, each of these short exercises is meant to connect your awareness back to your body and your way of being in the world. It's so easy to have all these vague hopes and fears that swirl around in our minds, but getting clear about them allows us to take the next steps forward and actually do something about them.

You know, I see how this might help me, but aren't there a lot of other things like food and exercise to deal with? I feel like I need to be starting my diet and hitting the gym right now.

Oh, you are right, but remember earlier when we talked about laying a foundation? This is important because it creates a strong structure for the "doing" part. The system you use to help you with the nutrition and exercise is important, too. We just want to be sure you can start the journey and then keep going for the rest of your life.

Whenever we commit to a new path, there will be some people who will cheer us on and do everything in their power to help us. There will be others who aren't crazy about what we are up to because they may feel badly about themselves and aren't ready to make the change themselves.

Right now I'd like you to get out your notebook and write this:

My Top Five Cheerleaders

These are people who will give you their wholehearted support. They want you to succeed and they will be thrilled to learn about your progress. You will know who they are because when you tell them you have committed to a whole new you, they will give you some version of a high five. These are the people who will not caution you, try to discourage you, tone you down, or remind you about your past attempts. Just the opposite is true of these people. They will support you, encourage you and even give you great ideas you hadn't considered before—some of them might even help you cook healthy, delicious food!

Remember that we said earlier how you will draw a line in the sand and commit to this process? Well, these are people you will recruit to be on your cheerleading squad. Please be sure to pick well.

Do you have those people's names in your notebook?

There's a chance that you might not be able to come up with five cheerleaders. That's okay. Write down one, three, four or ten. I asked for five because it's a solid number and shouldn't require too much thought, but even one really strong supporter can make all the difference. Also, as you move forward, you will meet new people who will gladly take on this role. You don't even know them yet, so stay tuned. The universe is ready to help you cross their paths at exactly the right time.

Going forward, I will give you simple ideas for how to get them on your team and help you stay honest.

Now let's take a look at the current habits you have that do not support your desire for a strong, healthy body.

Write a new heading in your notebook. You may want to start a new page for this, because you will begin to notice other things to add to the list as your awareness grows.

My Top Five Unsupportive Habits

These can be things like "come home after work and lie on the couch watching TV for hours", or "eat four bagels a day", or "drink beer every night to relax", to "I smoke cigarettes" —whatever you already know isn't helping you move into a place of joy in your body, but you just revert to out of habit.

Please write them down in short phrases. Remember, this doesn't need to take long. The quicker, the better. What's important here is clarity and honesty.

Also, you aren't committing to stop those habits just yet. At this point you are only turning on the lights so you can see what you've been stumbling over. If these are long-established patterns, it doesn't do much good to say, "I'll never do it again", just like it isn't smart to say, "I'll work out for two hours at the gym every day" when you haven't been exercising in years.

We want to identify the things that are there now, and this

isn't meant to cause you shame. Just the opposite is true, in fact. I want you to accept that these patterns have been part of your life. Human beings all use things to cope and we don't do ourselves any good by pretending we don't. Believe it or not, some people use exercise and diet in obsessive, unhealthy ways. You might look at them and see a fitness model picture of health, but some are just addicted to behaviors that make them look really good and are still a complete mess on the inside.

The process we are working through now is designed to launch you gently into a new way of behaving, moving, and eating—but it is also meant to feel natural, which means you can enjoy it and keep it up forever.

All of this sounds wonderful, but I have to say that I want to be realistic. I don't want to set up such a big transformation goal that I can't get there, or I fall down along the way because it's just too much to handle.

Just before the first chapter I shared the Taoist quote: *"A journey of a thousand miles begins with a single step."*

What I'd like you to do now is let yourself dream. Why don't we go there first and then I'll explain more about how to use the feeling of your dream to guide the steps in between?

Take your notebook and write this down:

My fitness dream is...

After that, spend five or ten minutes writing down exactly how you want your body to feel, what you want to be able to do, and even the kind of clothes—including size—you would just love to wear.

Powerful Self Talk Tip: Write this in the present tense and only in positive language. Example: *"My body is light, lean, and strong. I love feeling my muscles when I walk and I am getting stronger every day now. When I step out of the shower and see myself naked in the mirror, I love my reflection. I can go to the store and buy clothes right off the rack that fit perfectly..."*

Are you feeling this? It's really easy once you get into it, and you don't have to worry about anyone else reading this, so allow yourself to be as descriptive as you want. It's best if you can add some sensuous, sexy details to get your mind and body engaged. Again, this isn't for anyone else to see. This is your own dream. You own it and you don't have to explain or defend it to anyone.

After you have written out a word picture of yourself enjoying this body of yours, please close your eyes and take a couple of deep, slow breaths. Then read the words aloud and feel into what you have just set out as what you really want.

How does this feel?

I asked this question of a client recently and she said, "Well, it feels unrealistic."

We laughed together and then I said, "Thank you for being honest about that. Like moving into a brand new house or driving a new car for the first time, it is unfamiliar. You were really used to the old version—you knew where everything was and all the normal squeaks and rattles. You knew what didn't work and how to deal with that. This new vehicle doesn't feel 'real' yet and that's okay. It will take a little getting used to."

So, how do we use this faraway dream image to help us way back here where the journey begins?

I am reminded of the explorers in olden times when the world was younger and a lot of it hadn't been discovered yet. Many of them used maps that were wildly inaccurate and depicted fanciful landscapes and creatures that didn't exist, like dragons or great sea serpents. But they had a dream of what was possible out there. They believed they'd find gold and spices and wonderful lands. These visions kept them going through unimaginable hardships. Without the grand idea, they would have never begun.

You and I aren't plunging into wild, unknown seas, though. This path has been traveled by many before us. Of course, it is still foreign to us because we have yet to do the trip ourselves, but it isn't as if we are risking life and limb. We have all sorts of wonderful scientific information to guide us. We have trainers and teachers to show us what to do, how often to do it, and everything else we need.

What I'm offering is a way to connect to the feeling—the emotion—which is the real magic in the equation. As you make this commitment and then take the first steps on what may seem like a forever long journey, you need the emotion and the feeling of what you desire anchored in your body.

Robert Fritz wrote, *"If you limit your choice only to what seems possible or reasonable, you disconnect yourself from what you truly want, and all that is left is a compromise."*

We talked about it a little earlier, but it's worth revisiting. When you get truly clear on who you are, where you are now, and what you desire, you activate a mysterious set of serendipities and synchronicities that enter the picture to support your actions with the right people, information, and opportunities.

That's what we are doing here: getting clear.

Then we are taking that to the next level. We are feeling it. This is when we take an idea from the purely mental arena and bring it into our bodies.

The more we test drive, then take ownership of these new, inspiring feelings and thoughts, the easier it is to make them real in the physical world.

So, in terms of being realistic, it's good to be "unrealistic" and then work backward from there to find our feet exactly where they are right now.

The thoughts that I have shared in *Begin With Yes* and other books and CDs is really much more than a collection of happy thoughts. I know this is true, because they tell the story of my life. In the spirit of transparency, not every dream of mine has come true, but so many of them have. Some of you might remember that when I was a kid, I wanted to be a trapeze artist. Well, life did get in the way, but I've never totally given up on that picture in my head. Last Christmas I got a gift certificate for a trapeze lesson, so it looks like one day soon (I need to lose five more pounds to be under the weight limit) that dream will become a reality.

One other quick story about my book, *Begin With Yes*. Before I had written a single word, the book's title got planted in my head in such a powerful way that I just couldn't shake it. Within weeks, I had decided that title could become a book. So, I had to sit myself down, get a blank piece of paper and write the very first sentence.

If you are new at "thinking big thoughts" and taking small steps, your life as you know it is about to be transformed. *Begin With Yes* techniques work in just about every part of your life. Once you get the hang of it, making things happen will become second nature. So, I say yes! Write a book, fly the trapeze, meet new people, learn the piano, become a baker—or even get fit.

Okay, we keep talking about first steps. I'm anxious to get started. How do I take the first steps?

That itchy feeling is great. It means you are ready to take action. Now, we know that you aren't going to be content with just thinking about this, hoping for it, and putting it off.

Because we are still laying the foundation for all that action you will take, it may seem like we are sitting around talking and lifting nothing but a pen. It probably seems like none of this is going to burn any calories, doesn't it?

This reminds me of the story of a man who decided to climb Mt. Everest. He spent over a year researching and training for the big adventure—buying gear, reading books, and talking to everyone he could about mountaineering. When the time came to fly to Kathmandu and begin the actual climb, he was surprised to learn that it took the better part of two weeks just to get to the Base Camp. The trek across the long valley was exhausting all by itself. For days he didn't feel like he was actually climbing any mountains. He had read the books, talked to guides, and studied everything he could, but nothing could prepare him for reality of the long stretch before the real climb began. He finally expressed his frustration and one of his guides said, "You started climbing Mt. Everest before you ever left your home. Everything is part of the climb."

It is just that way for this process of transformation, too. Reading this book, doing the self discovery exercises, locating your resources and helpers, and visualizing your success are all critical steps.

In other words, you are already in motion.

As I have proved in my own life and watched so many readers and clients discover, the moment we take a firm, decisive step toward what we truly desire, things—amazing things—begin to happen. I love what Henry David Thoreau famously wrote: *"I learned this, at least, by my experiment: that if one advances confidently in the direction of his dreams, and endeavors to live the life which he has imagined, he will meet with a success unexpected in common hours."*

So, this might be a great time to take another step. Remember, you haven't drawn the line yet. You haven't stepped across it. This time is different. You are taking your time and discovering exactly what you want. You are also taking time to feel what the Zen Buddhists call "right action".

We live in a culture that demands constant action. We are pushed and pulled by the loud voices of advertising and competition and social pressures. As a result, we often take action that isn't aligned with our own needs and desires.

How often have you made a decision to read a book, join a gym, start a diet, or go to a movie simply because it seemed popular or appeared to offer a solution? I know I have done that many times. It's not bad, either. That's what humans do. We experience things and then we share those experiences with others. The trouble is that this started to become artificial when the age of modern advertising was born not long after World War II. With the advent of television, and the need to fund the production of all these new programs, came the companies who would pay to have their products mentioned. Pretty soon our minds were affected not so much by the simple endorsement of one friend to another saying, "you should try this…", but by the increasingly scientific and often manipulative advertising industry.

I'm not scolding our culture or even the advertisers, either. The modern world is full of wonderful products and ideas that we wouldn't have right now if it weren't for entrepreneurs finding ways to tell us about them through ads. I just want to invite you back into a natural, gentle process of finding out what you really want and what works best for you. That requires stepping back from the urgency of "sign up for this right now…just $99 for the next two days!", and only enroll in programs that fit your needs and your body best.

As you plan the next stage of this journey, I encourage you to ignore the shiny fitness magazines at the supermarket checkout stand. Instead, talk to some of your close friends who are doing well with their fitness. Ask them about their routines and the programs they use. Perhaps go sample yoga or use a day pass at their gym (which you can often get at no charge or much less than $20) and try out their spin class or a group "body pump" session. Maybe rent a bike and go cycling with some friends. This is a treasure hunt! You are finding out what works for you rather than just signing up for anything that comes along because you know you need to do something rather than nothing. You won't find just one thing that will cover every single one of your fitness needs and also keep you interested for a long time. That's why it is a good idea to just open yourself up to a lot more experiences and let yourself be drawn by the ones that feel good and are challenging in ways that inspire you.

Can you feel how this becomes fun? Instead of just jumping into a program because it is popular or someone is selling it, you are sampling, testing, and feeling. That starts to feel like wonder, play, and possibility, doesn't it?

Some of you may be wondering about my own experience

with getting healthier. I actually tried a few quick fixes that didn't deliver and then researched several programs before I settled on the "Commit To Get Fit" program at my gym. This program didn't promise an instant fix. It did promise that, if I did my part, it would change my life—and together we have proved that promise.

A few minutes ago you said, "I'm anxious to get started. How do I begin taking those first steps?"

Because you asked about how to start taking first steps, I wanted to offer some ideas about actually moving your body. If you go back to the Mt. Everest expedition story, think of these as training hikes. You aren't trekking into Base Camp quite yet, but you are definitely not just sitting on your couch looking at pictures of Kathmandu, either. You have begun and your actions backed by intent and desire have already activated the immense, intelligent matrix of the universe to serve up synchronistic information, guides, and resources that will help you make it all happen. I'm not even asking you to believe that this is true. Please feel free to doubt everything I'm saying—as long as you just take a step. I am confident that you will begin to experience these things for yourself, and when you do, it's not because I proved a point for myself. I share these things because they have changed my life and the lives of so many I have met along the way. It's too good not to share this with you.

I can't wait to get started now. This is an entirely different thing than I was imagining. It almost seems too easy or fun—like maybe it's not serious enough to make a difference.

Isn't it funny how we adults have forgotten how to make real magic? How many children do you know who lay out their day with checklists and get all serious about "project managing" their lives? Children in their natural state will go outside and play. They won't eat too much. They will jump and run and ride bikes. They will feel the simple joy of being themselves in their bodies—and come running inside before bed all tired and dirty.

We have made life too heavy. Is it any wonder that our bodies and minds and spirits get heavy? A lot of what I'm sharing with you in this conversation is the idea that we can lighten up and still get everything we want.

Don't worry, though. Before this discussion is over, I will

invite you to enter into a real contract with yourself so your rational mind will be comfortable that you are ready to make a change. In other words, I'll ask you to commit. If the program you've found doesn't ask you to make this kind of commitment, you will just have to do what the program's creator forgot, take matters into your own hands and make the commitment yourself.

For now, I want you to experience the amazing shift that occurs when we change our inner state from heaviness into lightness, from seriousness into play—then allow our bodies to experience the same things.

Our lives are created by beliefs. One of the beliefs I want to help you change is that change has to be hard or terribly painful. Certainly most of the big changes in our lives are accompanied by stretching and pressure. I'm sure you can look back and see where pain has been a teacher during those times and you probably learned a lot from the pain you experienced. But I want to introduce you to a new teacher. Her name is Joy.

What if you could take some classes taught by Joy? It's not as if most schools have only one classroom. Physical transformation isn't different in this way.

Sure, when you need to decide between sleeping in and getting up to exercise, or between eating something lean and nutritionally supportive rather than a juicy, greasy cheeseburger, it might not be comfortable at first. But is that really pain?

How we frame things in our minds—the story we tell ourselves about them—is so important. If we tell ourselves and everyone around us how hard it is, how sore our muscles are, how badly we want to quit, this keeps us in the Pain classroom.

What if we simply start focusing on the fact that we have taken new action and the new results are on their way? What if we started noticing everything that is working and all the tiny positive changes that start showing up, like the pants fitting just a little better or how delicious the lean chicken and quinoa salad is?

These are just a couple of examples, but if you can begin to really believe that Joy and Pleasure are also teachers, you will get results faster than you can probably handle.

Rather than repeating the mantra, "No Pain, No Gain", let me invite you to move in the direction of this quote: *"Respect your body. Eat well. Dance forever." — Eliza Gaynor Minden*

Why should it be any harder than that?

I'm also reminded of this beautiful piece of *The Desiderata*, a poem by Max Ehrmann wrote in 1927 that became wildly popular in the 70's:

Beyond a wholesome discipline, be gentle with yourself.
You are a child of the universe no less than the trees and the
stars;
you have a right to be here.

Be gentle with yourself.

Just like the trees and stars, we have a right to be here as ourselves. It is only our own artificial ideas about so many things that makes our journey through this world difficult. What if becoming everything you can possibly be in this lifetime is perfect and enough?

So, how do I find the power switch inside myself in those times when I feel weak and helpless?

You ask the best questions.

The truth is, we all have those times. Take a look around you at all the people you imagine never have a weak moment—never sit on the couch eating a whole pint of ice cream, hit the snooze button rather than getting up to exercise, or make some excuse rather than do the thing they know will move them closer to their desires—you will find that every one of us is human.

So what is the critical difference between those who seem to make things happen in their lives and those who are always only wishing for something better?

You know, it is a lot simpler than you might suspect.

The watershed moments in our lives are rarely the ones we

remember. They are the small steps, the most modest choices. It really does come down to that.

Here are some examples of baby step actions that can shift you into a whole different gear:

- Go to the store and buy a few "nutritionally supportive" items that you know you will eat.
- Get up, lace your shoes and take a walk around the block.
- Call the gym and ask when the next Spin Class takes place—then put it on your calendar.
- Find a friend and schedule a long walk followed by a healthy lunch at a restaurant you both enjoy.
- Walk into your kitchen and drink one or two tall glasses of water.

None of these seem like they will do very much toward your big goal of transformation, do they?

The truth is, though, when you are feeling powerless or

depressed about your progress, it is more important than ever to simply take an action in the direction of your desires.

Please remember that phrase: *in the direction of.* It is one of the most important in this entire book. If you can tattoo this in your awareness, you will have a critical key to unlock all the doors between here and where you want to go.

Picture a toaster. Yes, just like one you probably have on your counter right now. It has a cord and a plug. The only way it works is if you plug it into the wall socket. Now, imagine this socket with wires running behind your walls, under the ground and out to the street where they join the power grid. But it doesn't stop there. Miles and miles away, power station after power station connects this system to a nuclear power reactor with mind-boggling energy available twenty-four hours per day. You may use your toaster every day for something simple like browning a bagel or a piece of bread, but you are tapping into the immense power of this generator miles away.

That is what happens when you take a small step forward on days that feel heavy or dark. Instead of falling backward into all those old habits of coping, when you take a walk or drink plenty of water, you are sending a signal to your conscious and subconscious mind. You are making the statement that you have decided upon a certain course of action. When you do this, as Goethe said, "…mighty forces will come to your aid."

Those great and mighty forces are always there, just like the nuclear generator is always out there making more electricity. What you do when you take a small action is something like making the choice to plug your toaster into a wall socket. It seems insignificant, but that is because you can't see the billions of watts you have just tapped for your use.

Too often we assume that we need to take some quantum leap when what is really important for that moment is something that seems small. Johann Goethe wrote, *"Be bold and mighty forces will come to your aid."* I have always loved this thought. It rings a bell somewhere inside, doesn't it?

I hope you can understand that this part of our conversation—triggered by your question—is one of the most powerful parts of this little book. If you will accept that not only can this journey be gentle and joyful, but also comprised of many small, do-able steps, everything about it will be possible.

Did you know that if you exercise just 15-20 minutes per day, six days per week, you will achieve things most people think is impossible for themselves within less than a year? It is true. Small, consistent actions over time make all the difference, not the massive, painful exertions of weekend warriors who get into the gym and kill themselves for hours.

Access your "power switch" by remembering what you are plugging into when you move just a little bit every day toward what you desire most.

You used the words, "…when I feel so weak and helpless…" Those times are exactly when you can take the smallest, most believable actions. When you are full of power and energy, you can turn up the dial to eleven and have a lot of fun, but when you are low on willpower, just do something small in the right direction.

This is much like climbing a spiral staircase. Around and around we go. The choice we make every day is whether to move upward toward our desires or turn and go down into despair. I invite you to take just one step up today. If that feels great, maybe take two or three more—but take at least one step up every day. We can all do that, can't we? I'm going to drink a tall glass of water and stretch right now.

What I'd like to do now is ask you to tell me those other things on your mind. I want you to feel free to voice doubts or fears that make you wonder if you can really do it this time.

Well, okay. Here goes. I have been both wanting this and putting it off for a very long time. I can't tell you how many times I have said "I will start this coming Monday."

You know, this is so common. Much like writing this very book, in fact. I had it "on my list" for a few years, but life kept getting in the way. Don't feel bad about yourself or how many times you haven't started when you said you would.

No, I'm not just letting you off the hook to make you feel better. I'm reminding both of us that every major worthwhile thing we do seems big. Sometimes we just feel exhausted by the many little things we have to do every day. It doesn't always make sense when we step back from it. I mean, we don't have good, rational excuses—most of us aren't going through something intense like medical school, or something like that. If we add up the duties and activities of our days, almost all of us can find half an hour to exercise. As we talked about earlier, even just fifteen minutes, six days per week will work wonders. So, we can't come up with valid excuses, but here we are weeks, months, and years later with the book still lying around as scattered notes or the extra pounds hanging on our body.

Let's break that pattern now, shall we?

Get up. Yes, go ahead and get up right now. Put down this book or carry it with you. Either way is fine. Right now, go outside and take a walk around the block. If it's thirty below zero outside maybe walk the length of your hallway ten times quickly.

Go for it.

Are you back from that mini-workout now?

You just started. You just took steps forward. Whether today is Wednesday, Saturday or Monday, you didn't wait.

Now do the same thing tomorrow just to prove to yourself that you can do it and not put things off. I know this seems ridiculous, but it is an important signal to your subconscious mind.

Powerful Self Talk Tip: As you take these steps say this out loud, "I am moving NOW in the direction of my goals and dreams. Every step I take NOW gets me closer."

You are holding this finished book in your hands right now, so it probably seems different from what you are doing with your fitness—but it is very much the same. In this moment, I am sitting here typing one word at a time. I have so many other things to do: feed the dog, check Facebook for important messages that need response, send a text to the friend whose birthday I just remembered is today, get ready for dinner with my boyfriend, and too many others to even list here. It is so easy to talk myself out of sitting here and writing a few pages that will become the book you are now reading.

That's kind of mind bending, isn't it? You just time traveled back to where I haven't yet finished this book, so in a real way we are taking this journey together. Now, I am jumping forward in time to sit next to you and have this conversation about taking steps and writing words.

It is the only way to get things that matter to us done. Start right now, then keep going.

Right now I am having a wonderful image of you reading my finished book. That helps me write this next sentence.

Can you see how this works?

Hold the image of the body you want to create and see yourself enjoying that. Feel yourself taking a light jog, or going dancing, or making love in your new body. Then do the equivalent of writing this next sentence—go drink a glass of water and take a walk for ten minutes.

There's an old saying, "Life by the yard is hard, but by the inch it's a cinch." I think this fits in well here because we often use our minds to jump forward in the future and imagine the big job ahead of us rather than take the easy inch right at our feet. The best use of our mind's ability to project into the future is by creating an inspiring image of what we want, let that change the feeling in our body, then use that feeling as fuel to take action in this moment.

Here's something else, since you just had me get started now. I always start things off with a lot of positive, "can do" energy that typically lasts less than a week. I make a poor choice, miss a day at the gym, have a donut and then it just seems to unravel.

This is a good one. I'm glad you brought it up. With the exception of those few superhuman-seeming people who never start something without a fully laid out plan that they always stick to, most of us are much more excited about the beginnings of things.

There are good neurological reasons for this, too. At the beginning of exciting things, including falling in love, dopamine, a neurotransmitter (which, interestingly enough, is best known for its ability to initiate muscle movement) is triggered in our brains. Dopamine is triggered when we make a decision to move toward something we want. Marketing researchers have noticed that many people get a "dopamine high" just by clicking the "BUY" button or swiping their credit card if they feel that the new course, or gym membership, or some other exciting product will be a solution to their problems—especially if those problems are in the hot spot pain areas of health, money, or relationships.

Does this sound familiar?

Many people let the small rush of dopamine carry them into purchase after purchase over time while the new exercise bike, or running shoes, or ab flexer stays in its box, unused. How many times have you seen basically brand new fitness equipment at yard sales? Often you just got a bargain because the people who originally bought those items new were riding the dopamine wave and didn't know that, to keep the good feelings rolling, they needed to actually move their bodies!

So, dopamine is an important, natural chemical in our bodies that helps us get moving. The "natural high" effect fades fairly quickly. But, it can come back over and over again if we keep moving toward what we desire, because each time we achieve another goal and move into the quest for more, dopamine reinforces our good feelings about that.

However, we need to be aware that this can be a roller coaster ride that will leave us feeling depressed if we don't know how to manage it.

A lot of this gets attached to the definitions and labels we place on different actions. In other words, if you label *"Went to the gym"* as a huge win, you will get a positive effect by making that happen. On the other hand, if you label *"Ate a donut"* as a major crime against yourself, it will reinforce the idea that you really can't do this and, once again, you are "headed for failure so why try anyway?"

Now, if you eat two or three donuts every day, you may not make the progress you want with your weight loss goals. It is good to be honest about these things; however, if you eat a donut some morning, it isn't the end of the world. If you can help yourself place less negative weight on a single action like this and remember that, in the bigger picture, it doesn't mean anything about your ability to keep advancing steadily and gently. Also, an average donut has approximately 195 calories. In an entire day's worth of eating, that isn't much. Even if you are on a reduced-calorie plan, that isn't going to blow you out of the water.

Again, I'm not trying to give you a bunch of easy outs. It is just that I feel it is important to keep things in perspective because our minds are expert at crafting disaster scenarios over relatively minor facts.

I hope this demystifies the stop-start, fall-off-the-wagon cycle that can be so discouraging if we allow it to define us as weak or unable to finish what we start.

Making a long term goal and then keeping a sense of humor about our own humanity as we move toward it will help a lot.

That reminds me again of what we said earlier—*"Progress, not perfection."* This reminder can help us if we get an inch or two off the path. If we eat a cheeseburger when that's not part of the plan, or drink too many glasses of wine at a friend's party, the best thing to do is chuckle and move right back into the commitment we have made to the journey. Eat a 1,200 calorie cheeseburger and you have a couple of days' worth of adjustment to make. Eat a cheeseburger every day for two weeks and you have probably set yourself back further than some would have wished—but even then, the solution is the same. The key is to notice where you stepped backward and just take a few simple steps forward.

Also, be careful about enrolling in any plan that requires absolutely rigid adherence with no days off. The human psyche is such that we all need rewards and breaks. Without them, we can unconsciously become rebellious and start behaving in counterproductive ways without even knowing why. I suggest that you choose a system that helps you modify most of your behavior but leaves room for being human.

I kind of hate to admit this, but I actually don't like the foods I am supposed to eat.

You made me chuckle because it's one of the first questions I was asked in my own "Commit To Get Fit" program. The truth is, we live in a world that has conditioned us to want foods that are not really good for us. None of us should feel badly about this. It is just a result of how humanity has evolved over these many millions years. Several hundred years ago we wouldn't be having this discussion. We would be working much too hard to obtain the bare minimum of food we need to survive.

What we have now is a result of all the amazing progress we have made as the human race. Sometime in the 1900's, we began producing most of our food in factories and selling it in stores rather than growing it ourselves or purchasing it from neighboring farmers. In those days, everything we ate was "organic". Now we pay extra for that label and sometimes it's not clear whether or not we're getting what we paid for.

Now, this doesn't help much with the statement you just made. I just want you to know that it is something all of us must deal with. It's a problem of choice.

In the past we had very little choice. Now when you go to the condiments aisle, you are faced with an array of at least dozens of salad dressings—all of which have varying calorie counts, fat content, and other things to consider.

In other words, we have a lot of choices these days. Rather than complain about that, I want to invite you to play with it. Pretend that you are a king sitting on a throne. You are bored with everything, since you can have literally anything you desire. Now all you want is the best or purest of what's available.

Next time you walk through the grocery store, play this out in your mind. Pretend you have a scepter and you only accept the things that will be both delicious and nutritionally supportive. I won't try to give you a list of things to eat in this book. If you have chosen a good system or a good health coach, they will guide you to learn what is best for you.

The important thing is to start to shift your beliefs about what is "good for me". Just because it's obvious that celery is a low calorie choice doesn't meant that it is the only one you can select. In fact, you will be shocked to learn how many foods contain low or even negative calories (meaning that you burn more calories digesting them than they add to your overall diet). Do a simple Google search on "Negative Calorie Foods" and amaze yourself at how many choices you have. Did you know that you can design a daily menu plan that will include foods you like and leave you feeling stuffed? You absolutely do not have to starve yourself to make this work—just the opposite is true. You can focus on foods that make you feel great, taste wonderful, and help you reach your goals quickly.

The human psyche is such that none of us likes to feel overly restricted. We want choices. So, give yourself a lot of them.

The really good news is that there are so many that you will find both delightful and healthy.

I was surprised to learn this after I committed to my own fitness transformation. Basically, I had fallen into patterns of eating certain things and those well-worn habits made me believe that I only wanted those foods. When I started exploring, I discovered that there were so many options outside of my usual fare that I almost couldn't keep track. Not all of these required me to do a lot of planning or preparation, either. I travel often and lead a very busy schedule. I eat at restaurants frequently and deal with all the usual stress of modern living. When I made the commitment to change, I discovered that there were whole sections of the menu I hadn't noticed for years.

Even if you are working with a tight budget, you will find that the Internet is packed with recipes and suggestions that will help you make eating easy, filling and even fun.

As I teach in my first book, *Begin With Yes*, nothing is more important than making the decision for change. Once you have done this, circumstances and opportunities seem to arrange themselves around your powerful intent much more easily than you first imagine.

Here's something else. I encourage you to learn all you can about "real food" versus "diet food". If you use a strong plan to build a new menu for yourself and make sure it consists of real food, you will find that your body and your appetite both begin to change. Before long, you will clean up the old way of eating and your body will crave more of what is making it feel so good.

Have you ever drank a delicious green smoothie with lots of amazing ingredients and felt your body say "yes!"? Maybe you have had that experience with some kind of wholesome salad loaded with arugula and spinach and other high-energy ingredients? There's this moment after you are full of truly good, nutritious food when your body sends out all sorts of "thank you signals". That's your body saying YES.

The more you help your body say "yes" to real food—the kind of food that feeds your cells with exactly what they need to be electrified by healthy energy—you will discover that you will never need to say "no" again. Because the better you feel, the more of that feeling you want. Before long, when you have a day off and eat a big slice of pizza or a pulled pork sandwich, you will notice that you just don't want as much of it as you once would have. Sure, it's nice to eat some of those wonderful things, but you might even discover that once you get your system tuned up, you don't feel great when you put poor quality fuel in it.

I hate to sound like a whiner, but the truth is that my family is not helping me. They haven't been on board with my new fitness plans in the past, and I have no reason to believe they will be now. What should I do about this?

I'm glad you brought this up. This is a big deal and we can't afford to gloss over it. Families are the best—and the worst. They can be our biggest cheerleader squad, and they might be mired in patterns that they aren't excited to change. Any time someone in a particular "tribe" makes a break with the usual way of doing things, they are often faced with resistance.

Have you ever told your friends that you were going to quit drinking, stop smoking, move to a different city, or go back to college? Did you notice that a few were extremely supportive while most of them gave you reasons why it might not work?

Families are no different, except we usually have the deepest attachment to their opinions. This is normal. We share DNA with them—which means we also share old family patterns, habits and beliefs. One of the most powerful forces in human nature is to remain consistent with who we believe ourselves to be. We can't change the family into which we were born, even though we might not agree with their ideas or lifestyles anymore.

I suggest that as you work through this process of commitment to yourself, you will identify people inside your family and also outside supporters who will help you keep going. I have had many clients tell me, "No one in my family has ever done this before". If that describes you, don't despair. This doesn't mean you have to alienate everyone at Thanksgiving Dinner.

It is surprising to discover that you can actually break from tradition without conflict. You can still sit down with everyone for a meal but only put things on your plate that you know will be satisfying and keep you on track with your most important desires.

Isn't it funny how we assume that others will judge us for eating a smaller portion of mashed potatoes and gravy? If we just go quietly about our business, they will probably not even notice. The problem often arises when we feel that we must become the new fitness evangelists and make everyone around us change.

The best preaching we can ever do is by living our own truth. When you show up to the next family gathering looking wonderful in your new, smaller clothes, it makes much more impact than all the speeches you might make at the table about how everyone should start eating better.

The bottom line is that change is uncomfortable—especially for those who aren't ready for it themselves. I encourage you to find a supportive, like-minded community of people who are committed to the same kind of transformation you desire. Don't even worry about close friends or family members who haven't decided to do this for themselves. If you simply love them just as they are, where they are, you won't find yourself in so much conflict with them as you make your metamorphosis.

The truth is, I don't have much of a support system. My friends aren't any healthier than I am and I am not sure where to look for or find encouragement. Any ideas?

Well, we just discussed the family dynamic, but our circle of friends is pretty close to the same situation. Some of us haven't lived near our families for a long time, so our close associates are even more important in terms of how we live from day to day.

As I suggested a minute ago, I encourage you to find a "tribe" of people who are committed to the same transformation as you. Because you are all leaning into the same goals and dealing with similar challenges, you will have a lot to talk about. This turns out to be one of the critical issues. We need to be understood! If all of our friends are spending their weekends at sports bars eating French fries and nachos, it's easy to feel like the odd person in the mix when we order healthier choices. On the other hand, if you find a group of people who love to hike, walk, or ride bikes and then find a place to hang out and chat over just one beer, it makes things a lot easier.

I talked about this in my first book, *Begin With Yes*. I never want to suggest alienating friends and family, but when you begin to make choices for yourself, it is possible that some people will no longer fit in your close circle. Rather than suffer the loneliness of losing friends, I recommend adding new ones who are already of like mind with your new direction. It's possible that you will have to make some difficult choices, but in my experience, this isn't something you have to force at this point. Most people who aren't excited about your new direction will start to fade when you demonstrate that you are firm about what matters most to you. Something powerful happens when you begin to move in new circles. You make new friends, you feel good, and you attract more of what you need to support your choices.

In a lot of ways, I can see that this comes down to a different attitude that will help me take different actions from before. Is that what you're saying?

Yes. You just made me say my favorite word, by the way— "yes". Thank you. Attitude is critical.

This reminds me of a guy I often see at the gym...

A few days ago I asked him how he was, and his answer really summed up his reality in two words.

He said, "Mondays suck!"

At first I thought WOW, this would be a great story to tell, but then it occurred to me how sad this really was.

Because we're not talking about just one day

- We're talking about 52 Mondays a year that suck.

- If he lives to be 75, that's 3,900 days that suck
- If you do the math, that adds up over 10 years of this man's life ruined by a thought.

And don't you wonder what his Mondays would have been like if his thought was: "Mondays are a blessing – a chance to begin again and make something good happen"?

Well, all that to say, let's not be like the man in the gym. Let's remember that our thoughts are powerful because we're not only thinking them. We're believing them too.

What we believe, we take action upon. So, if we believe negative things about our bodies, our lives, our abilities, our families, or our friends, we are setting ourselves up to sabotage our best intentions.

I hope you can sense that I'm not asking you to splash a bucket of sunshine paint all over everything. We have been having a very honest conversation about the challenges and fears you may have about the process of transformation.

What I'm getting at with this part about attitude is that we can either face those obstacles with a "yes" attitude, or we can show up with an attitude that is weighted down with lots of heavy ideas. Why would we want to make it harder for ourselves?

Please don't blindly believe what I am sharing with you. Test these things for yourself.

You will know the feeling when it shows up to challenge you. In fact, let's go there now, shall we? Think back to a time when you were determined to accomplish something. You had made the decision, paid the money, bought the clothes, and were all ready to get started. Then someone came along and said a single negative thing. All of a sudden, what seemed so exciting and possible melted into a discouraging puddle at your feet. Can you remember a moment like that—maybe even a lot of them?

Did you feel…

- Deflated
- Discouraged
- Depressed
- Resentful
- Weak

If so, don't worry. That's normal.

What I invite you to do isn't normal. It interrupts those old stories of "this is how things go for me."

As you make this new commitment to yourself, you are going to know in advance that those challenges will show up. The difference is, you are preparing yourself to deal with them at this very moment.

It reminds me of some mythical tale when a hero goes out on an epic adventure, but just before she leaves, the magical helper shows up to give her a special sword or a bottle of powerful elixir or a tiny silver trumpet she can use in times of extreme need. That's what we're doing now.

We aren't ignoring the fact that the dragons and dark knights will show up during the journey. Of course they will! That's what makes it an adventure.

The difference is, your power object is your own desire and will to go all the way through. Armed with that and the shield of "yes" attitude, you now have protection against what has brought you down in the past.

Even framing this as an adventure helps, doesn't it? It means that we know up front that there will be highs and lows. There will be some dangerous valleys and rivers to cross. There is also a shining reward that makes the whole thing worth it. Can you feel that?

Oh, I can feel it. Right now I'm picturing myself looking and feeling like a whole new person—years younger and pounds lighter. I guess I want to know how I can find a balance between realistic, achievable goals and my dream body?

Well, it is good to be both a dreamer and a realist. At the same time. Picture your dream body. Feel yourself in it. Ah, isn't that amazing?

I talked with a friend recently who was finally able to go buy a pair of pants the same size he wore in high school. I asked him when he started the process if he knew he could go all the way back to that size.

He said, "I didn't even dare to dream that big at first. Of course, I had that idea hanging around, but it seemed like a completely unrealistic goal."

"So how did you do it?" I said.

He smiled and said, "I never tossed that dream. I made a goal of four sizes smaller than where I started. I could believe that! After a few months, I was buying those clothes and had so much more energy. I believed in myself like I hadn't for years. It wasn't such a stretch to imagine that I would have the willpower to keep going further. Plus, I was having so much fun and getting so many compliments that I had no desire to stop."

Exactly.

The rational mind always wants to put up "realistic" barriers. Rather than fight that, just move with it. Go ahead and say, "I will make my next big milestone wearing this size" or "I will weigh this many pounds". Do the believable and then gauge how you feel. I guarantee you that the positive feedback loops will be much stronger by then. This just means that your mind will have stretched and your energy will have increased. The next stage of the trip won't seem so long and you'll feel much better about it, too.

You say begin by loving my body as it is. That's easy to say but you haven't seen my body. When I stand in front of the mirror naked I am not one bit happy.

Now you're getting into real talk. There are so few people who love what they see in the mirror—even gorgeous celebrities who stay on the razor thin edge of physical beauty at all times struggle with self love and acceptance.

I saw something funny the other day. Here it is…

How To Be Skinny

Step 1: Notice that your body is covered in skin.
Step 2: Say, "Wow, I'm skinny!"

Congratulations, you are now skinny!

I hope you get a chuckle out of that, and it also illustrates a point. We constantly compare our shape and size to others.

As a result, we always feel anxiety about our bodies, and mostly at a subconscious level. If we see someone to whom we compare favorably, we might get a secret moment of satisfaction that "hey, I look pretty good" or "well, at least I'm doing better than they are." When someone shows up looking much better than we do, this quiet, critical voice starts saying things to us like, "you really have let yourself go" or "why don't I have enough discipline to get into that kind of shape?"

These reactions stay mostly hidden below the surface, but they run the show. They sabotage our ability to love ourselves and to make change for our own reasons.

So, what should we do about this situation?

I invite you to find a room in your house with a mirror where you can be completely private and practice something. Go there once per day, take all of your clothes off and just stand looking into your own eyes. Don't do an assessment or pinch that roll of fat around your midsection and frown. Just stare into your own eyes. Say, "I love you". Then say it again. Say it again, even if you don't feel the truth yet. Smile right into your own eyes. Take some time to remember that you have lived on this planet in your body for years—probably decades. This body-house of yours has moved around and helped you experience the world; touching, tasting, smelling, hearing, and seeing. How many challenges have you overcome while you've lived inside your own skin? The "You who is you" is a powerful, creative, dynamic creature that has been through a lot already. Take time to let yourself feel the truth of this and then say, "Thank you. I love you so much" to yourself at least once more with a smile.

Now this may feel fake or uncomfortable at first, but so do many things that we eventually master. This is no different. We need to master our response to life with, "I love you". Please do this once per day and just notice how it feels each day.

When you notice yourself having an unloving thought about yourself during your everyday busyness, take a moment to breathe and say "I love you". That's all. You don't have to excuse yourself or try to explain any behavior. Just offering yourself love over and over again will eventually challenge and then erase those old tapes, replacing the hurtful inner voices with one that is much more supportive and honest.

Again, I am not giving you a bunch of soft soap easy outs with this. You do want to transform and making changes in your body is part of that, but change begins within. How can we expect the world to be more supportive of us than we are to ourselves?

Are you willing to commit to this step of real mastery? If your answer is yes, then you have made a big leap forward, and it will change much more than just your own self talk. When you begin to speak to yourself with love, you will become kinder and more tolerant in other areas of your life. As this happens, you will notice how the outer world of other people and circumstances begins to mirror your inner transformation. Your body can't help but respond to this new attitude that you have toward it. You will become more comfortable in your own skin and you will also notice that you have much more power to change whatever you wish— one loving, gentle step at a time.

You know, I like the way you are teaching me to focus on small steps, but my class reunion is only 8 weeks away and I don't think the small steps are going to get me into the pants I was hoping to wear.

Talking about this now comes at a good time. Just after we chatted about loving the body we're in starting now. I'm glad you brought it up.

There are two things to think about here—and both of them are good:

One, having an impending reunion or wedding or some other event can be a wonderful way to stoke your commitment fire and help you start off with a lot of momentum. I have no problem with using upcoming events as stretch goals. That can add some extra fun and suspense to the game. If you are only trying to crash diet into a smaller pair of pants so you can look great at your reunion, you're probably entering a danger zone that will make it easy to slack off as soon as the meeting with your old friends is over. Since you are making a life long commitment to yourself, go ahead and sprint for the next eight weeks. Ask your trainer or check out the fitness plan you are using. Be willing to get laser focused and maybe a little crazy about it for this short period of time. Then when you come back home, step right back into the sustainable pace.

Two, I want you to be armed with extra self appreciation when you mingle with these people you haven't seen for a long time. As we just talked about, all the compliments or envious glances you might get can never replace your own love and self respect. Remember that all of the people you will see at the reunion have changed over time; it will help you keep the whole experience in perspective. Even the beauty queen who still has her hot little figure is probably worried about a few wrinkles or gray hairs. Imagine yourself spending the next eight weeks eating well and doing the exercises that are part of your plan. Two months may not be enough to put you back into your high school sized pants, but if you are fully committed to your own transformation, you will show up glowing with self respect and good energy. You may be surprised by how many people say, "You look great! What are you doing?" Even if you haven't lost that much weight yet.

That's what I want to keep bringing this back to—your commitment to yourself. It's funny, isn't it? When you asked that question, I went right into how to go ahead and work toward the result. There is absolutely nothing wrong with wanting to appear well in the eyes of others. That's the way we humans work, but it is only when we have a greater commitment to our own life, our own truth, and our own values that we will be able to get and keep the long term results we desire so much. This question flips backward on itself and leads us right here where we are at the moment; this place of decision.

Before we start talking about that, though, I do want to mention this thing of preferences. Sometimes we beat ourselves up for what we think is pure vanity.

Maybe you've heard someone say, "Well, I would get all fitness crazy and lose weight, but who am I kidding? At my age I don't need to impress anyone and that's just a bunch of fake vanity anyway."

Does this maybe sound like one of the voices in your head at times?

I would love it if you could come sit by me for a minute and let's just remember that there is nothing wrong with preference. It would be good for us to put down all of those judging thoughts about ourselves and just be okay with the fact that we would prefer to look and feel amazing.

Can you see how those voices get into battle and make us a little crazy? One voice says, "Until you lose all the weight, you'll never be good enough." The other says, "You have no business dreaming that big. Who are you to want to be beautiful? You think you're some kind of movie star or something?"

Earlier in our conversation, I asked you to write down your dreams of how you really want to look and feel. I encourage you to go back there and spend some time with those dreams again now. Maybe even build them out some more and upgrade a few of them.

I love everything you have been telling me, but I have to say that I deal with a disability and chronic pain, which makes it hard to imagine that I can be healthy. Can I still do this?

First, let me say how much respect I have for your courage to wake up every morning and face life. I know that the simple process of living is more challenging for you than for those who rarely experience anything more than a sore back or a headache.

If you have some issue that makes a "normal" exercise routine difficult or impossible, it is a good idea to spend time with a professional who specializes in these areas. After I wrote Begin With Yes, I began to connect with many thousands of people. Some of them have real life challenges that require expert assistance in addition to the process of becoming open to a "yes" way of life. For many, even taking that step forward has led to powerful new ways of getting much more of what they want in life—just scheduling an appointment or reading a book that deals with their specific needs is often that first step toward something much better.

Remember my personal story about wanting to be a trapeze artist when I was a child? Well here I am now, in my sixties, and there are many valid reasons to never revive that old dream. One thing that has helped me a lot is to focus on the feeling of what I desired back then. What did I want to feel as a trapeze artist? I have learned that I can still move toward the quality of that desire, and I have been amazed at how fulfilling it is to capture the essence of what I was after, even though I may never perform with Cirque du Soleil.

This is in no way an attempt to give you some glib answer. I only ask you to engage your powerful, creative mind and spirit and imagine how it is you want to feel. If you can take some specialized, specific steps toward those feelings, it may amaze you how many other possibilities rise to support your progress.

You have helped dig into so many things that always held me back in the past. I would like to talk about all of this forever, but I'm starting to feel like I might be stalling if I ask more questions right now. I think it might be time to make this commitment to myself.

We have been doing this for awhile, haven't we? It is one of my great joys to sit with someone who knows for sure that they want to move in a new direction and use conversation to reveal what is most important—and also the hidden fears or blocks that must be addressed for this to be possible.

As you just said, though, there is a time for talk and there is a time to take everything that has been said and use it for inspired action.

There are a couple of components here. The first is fairly straight forward. This is the "What". In other words, what are you going to use as a structure to help you achieve this wonderful new result in your life?

Earlier we talked about finding a particular practice or system that fits you really well. Ideally, this should be something that includes a few things.

Clear, do-able routines — You should be able to get involved with your new system without feeling completely overwhelmed by complicated instructions that are hard to maintain when you are not under the direct supervision of an instructor. You want to be able to take your practice with you at home, on the road, or wherever you find yourself.

Accountability — I highly recommend that you find a system that includes a group element if possible. There's something about knowing that other people expect you to show up and do something that makes it harder to quit or make excuses. How often have you showered, dressed and gone to a social engagement when you would have found some reason to stay on the couch, and afterward felt happy that you got out of your shell? It's much the same with having a group accountability system. You can also plug into some fine programs online that include a social component.

These keep things fun, accountable and include just a little competition to make it interesting.

Focus on Nutrition — As we discussed earlier, 80% - 90% of your results are directly affected by what you eat. This means that it is so important to find a system that helps you work out a healthy, sustainable plan for eating.

Stress Reduction — This is a critical aspect. Whatever plan you choose, please be sure it is one that helps you discharge nervous energy and anxiety from your mind and body. If the very thought of going to the next session stresses you out, it probably isn't the kind of system that will keep you engaged for the long term. It becomes too easy to start making excuses to avoid something that causes us stress. After all, we already have excessive stress in our busy lives and our plan for healthy living should help us reduce that, not cause more of it.

Fun — Sure, there are aspects of exercise that may not always feel like a party, but if this is going to work for you long-term, what you choose needs to include things you enjoy doing—or at least that you can learn to enjoy doing.

This isn't the definitive list of characteristics but it will give you a good place to start. I also know that we change and evolve. Don't worry about finding something that you are sure you will do for the rest of your life. If you can select one simple, effective core program to help you get on the right track, over time you will probably add other things like hiking, yoga, dancing, or swimming. You might find yourself attracted to join a bicycling group or adding long nature walks to the basic structure you use.

My main point is that we all need something that works simply, and to which we can return if we find ourselves getting off track some time in the future.

But before you sign on the line with any trainer or program, let's spend some time on the truest inner commitment—the only one, in fact, that will carry you through the entire journey.

I am asking you right now to make a rock solid commitment to just one person: you.

I suggest that you take some time and go back through the notes and exercises you have done during our time together. You might find one or two that you skipped over or to which you didn't give enough attention. If that's the case, now would be a good time to complete them. You are not doing this for me or because someone is going to give you a grade. This isn't homework! It is honoring yourself and your desires enough to do the inner work that prepares you for this next big step.

Think of it as pre-marital counseling in the best possible way. You are being honest with yourself about what you really want, what is important to you, what you fear, and what your previous disappointments or weaknesses have been.

Once you do this review and feel clear, I am going to invite you to marry yourself. I know that sounds odd, but think about it. Those of us who have been married know that we promise to "love, honor and cherish until death do us part." Many of us have also experienced a divorce, that means we, for whatever reason, couldn't keep that promise.

This one is different. You actually can vow to love, honor and cherish your body until death do you part. You are the only one to whom you can make that commitment with absolute confidence, and it this is the only "marriage" in which the choices of just one person dictate how happy and long-lasting it is. The truth is, you will live with your body until you die no matter what. This commitment you are making now is that your marriage to yourself will be joyful, supportive and fulfilling.

By the way, I am quite aware that many people have never married. Some have never had that desire and others have not been allowed to, until recently, because of outdated laws. If this describes you and you have trouble connecting with this idea, just imagine some partnership that is completely supportive on every level. Let yourself feel into what it would mean to have a healthy, honest connection. This could be in business, friendship, or some other intimate association in which two people need each other and can be of service to each other.

Because I am using this metaphor of a marriage, I'd like you to think about what it means to be in a conscious relationship with your body. Most of us spend a lifetime largely unconscious of how we live in these bodies. Now you are entering into vows with yourself, which means that even if you get off track sometime in the future, you are willing to be honest about it and find a way back into a loving, healthy relationship.

Can you see how different this is from some 90-day blitz? There's nothing wrong with an exciting blast to help things along, especially if you are the type of person who enjoys that, but this means making yourself and your health the Number One priority. For many of us, this will probably be the first time we have ever made that kind of promise in our lives.

Please, do take some time and go back over the ground we have covered. When you are ready, I want to offer a short commitment ceremony. It is one that you can perform all by yourself, or you can include some friends and supporters if you wish.

This is where you draw a line in the sand and then step across it into a new way of loving yourself.

Okay, I have given this a lot of thought. I am ready to commit. What do I do next?

At this point, I encourage you to do something different than you may have ever done for yourself before. I would like you to design a special ceremony for yourself to signify your commitment to this transformation of healthy, vibrant living.

We have many ceremonies in life. We graduate from kindergarten and high school. Some people have bar mitzvahs or bat mitzvahs. We get married, we get sworn in to the military or the legal profession, or take the Hippocratic Oath to become doctors.

In other words, our lives are full of ceremonies and they are almost always customs that have been designed for us by others. Ceremonies help us know that something has happened—a line has been crossed into a new way of living, working, or behaving. Often, once we have completed one of these rites of passage, we are given a new title of some kind, such as Mr., Mrs., Dr., Esq., etc.

What's interesting to me is how few of us have ever made up a ceremony all on our own to make something especially important.

Famous author and transformation coach Tony Robbins said, *"The most powerful force in the human psyche is people's need for their words and actions to stay consistent with their identity – how we define ourselves."* When we step across a line, sign our name to an important document, or raise our hand and pledge an oath, we have moved into a new version of ourselves. This cements something deep in our consciousness that we will then work very hard to maintain.

For example, most immigrants from others countries who go through the process of naturalization and become American citizens develop a tremendous sense of pride and responsibility that comes along with their title. They vote, start businesses, go to college, and work hard to take advantage of all the opportunities allowed by their new identity.

That is what I want you to do now. I want you to go through the internal process of accepting the fact that you have a strong, fit, healthy spirit and it is one that can move your body along into more of those things for itself, too. Sure, you may still be carrying some extra pounds at the moment, but you have that strong, vibrant self inside there. When you let that self know that you are committed to letting it come out, you better believe it will do everything in its power to help you accomplish it.

Can you feel the difference between that self-concept and the one that believes it is destined to be overweight, stressed out and lacking energy? Those two deeply held beliefs will each lead to a different set of behaviors to prove the truth of their position.

What we want to do now is to make a loving statement of release for an old way of being and fully embrace the truth of this new, healthy you that lives inside.

As far as how to do this is concerned, I encourage you to use your imagination and design a private ceremony that befits a major step forward. I will offer an example here in case you need a place to start, but please feel free to do whatever inspires you most.

The Commitment Ceremony

Set the stage by performing this in a clean, attractive space. Take a shower or bath and dress in clothes you feel good about wearing. Light a candle or two, and play music that inspires you.

If you feel most comfortable doing this alone, that's okay. It can increase the significance of the ceremony if you bring in someone you trust and who completely supports you as your witness.

You may wish to write this up, print it out, and read it aloud. Be sure to include your name in the blanks:

I, _____, have lived through a lot in this body. I take this time to thank myself and my body for carrying me through life so far. I have enjoyed so much good food and so many interesting experiences. My body is a map of the journey that I have taken to this point. I now enter a new era. I hereby vow to myself that, for the rest of my life, I will allow my body to become strong, healthy, and full of energy so that I may enjoy everything I wish to experience.

I, _____, am a powerful, dedicated person. I promise to feed my body with food that nourishes it, and my mind with ideas that inspire and strengthen it. I will exercise and play in my body so that it will feel and perform at its best.

I, _____, have a strong, fit, healthy spirit. I have stepped across this threshold into a new way of seeing myself and a new way of being in the world.

I know that this journey is meant to last for my lifetime. I am patient and gentle with myself as I transform and change. I embrace each day with the knowledge that I have the power to choose, and I now choose a life of joy and health.

Signed:

_____

Witnessed:

_____

Date:

_____

I have offered you this example and feel free to use it; however, it will become even more personal and powerful if you add your own words and feelings to it.

The main idea here is to create a moment in time that marks your commitment to yourself in a new way. If you do this with positive emotion, you will anchor it as a point of reference that you can look to whenever you feel you have strayed off course a bit.

My dearest hope is that you will join me and so many others who have chosen to create health, joy and freedom in their physical bodies and their lives.

Are you ready to begin now?

With sincere love and all best wishes for your journey ahead,

Paul Boynton
Optimist In Chief
Begin With Yes

About the Author

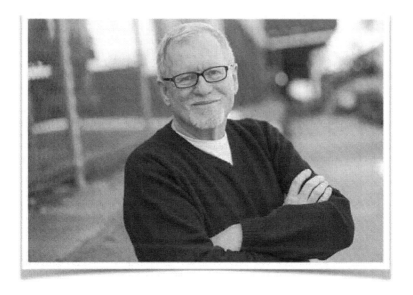

Paul Boynton *is the President & CEO of The Moore Center. He also blogs for The Huffington Post and The Good Men's Project, is a columnist for the NH Business Review and the host of "Begin with Yes" on Empower Radio. He is the author of several books including "Begin with Yes". His Facebook community, which has over a million followers is a source of inspiration for those who are taking steps toward a more meaningful life. You can read more at* www.beginwithyes.com *or on Facebook at* www.Facebook.com/beginwithyes

More books by Paul S. Boynton

Find these books and more by this author at Amazon.com

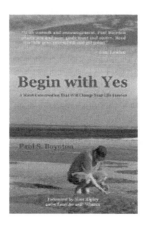

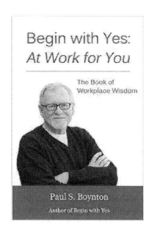

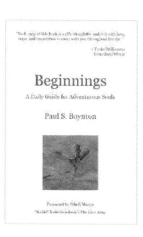

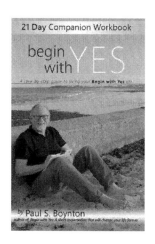

Join Paul Boynton and over a million Begin With Yes friends from around the world on Facebook!

www.Facebook.com/BeginWithYes

Visit the author at his website and subscribe for email updates
& inspiring newsletters

www.BeginWithYes.com

If you love this book and want to help others find it, please take a moment and post a review on Amazon. Thank you!